The Vibrant Lean & Green Dinner Cookbook

Tasty Lean & Green Dinner Recipes To Lose Weight

Jesse Cohen

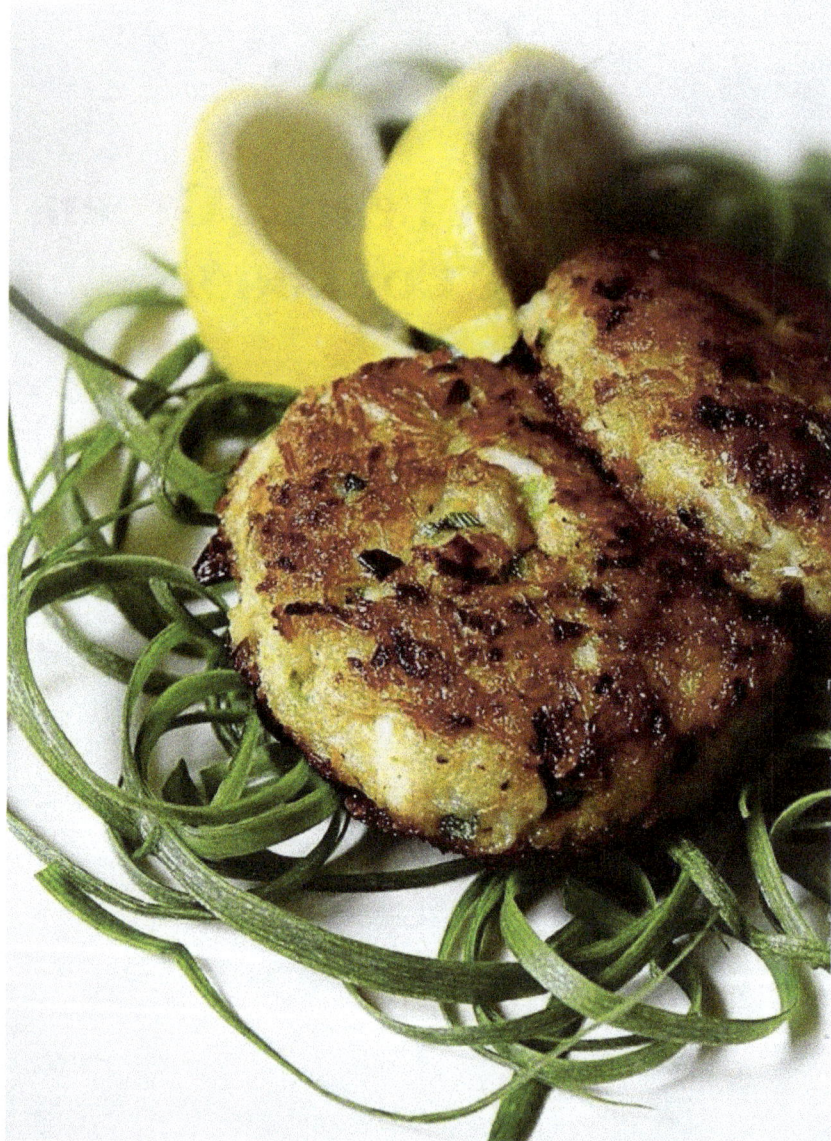

Table of contents

Super Tasty Onion Petals

Preparation time: 10 minutes

Cooking time: 15 minutes

Servings: 4

Ingredients

- 13 oz. of onion; peeled
- 1 teaspoon of basil; dried
- 1 teaspoon of ground coriander
- 1 tablespoon of olive oil
- ¼ teaspoon of ground nutmeg
- ¾ teaspoon of turmeric

Directions:

1. Cut the onion into the petals and sprinkle with the basil, ground coriander, olive oil, ground nutmeg, and turmeric.
2. Mix the onion petals and transfer them to the air fryer basket.
3. Cook the petals for 15 minutes at 375° F. Stir the petals every 3 minutes.

4. When the onion petals are cooked, they're going to have a soft texture.

5. Serve the entremots immediately!

Nutrition:

- Calories: 69
- Fat: 3.7 g
- Fiber: 2.1 g
- Carbs: 9 g
- Protein: 1 g

Eggplant Garlic Salad with Tomatoes

Preparation time: 10 minutes

Cooking time: 15 minutes

Servings: 6

Ingredients:

- 3 tomatoes; chopped
- 2 eggplants; chopped
- 1 tablespoon of olive oil
- 1 teaspoon of avocado oil
- 1 tablespoon of vinegar
- ½ teaspoon of ground black pepper
- ½ teaspoon of dried basil
- 2 garlic cloves; chopped

Directions:

1. Place the chopped eggplants in the air fryer.
2. Sprinkle the eggplants with the olive oil, ground black pepper, and dried basil.

3. Stir the eggplants and cook for 15 minutes at 390° F. Stir the vegetables every 5 minutes.
4. Then place the tomatoes in the bowl.
5. Add cooked eggplants, vinegar, and chopped garlic.
6. Then sprinkle the salad with the avocado oil and stir it.
7. Serve the cooked salad or keep it in the fridge!

Nutrition:

- Calories 80
- Fat: 2.9 g
- Fiber: 7.3 g
- Carbs: 13.6 g
- Protein: 2.4 g

Curry Eggplants

Preparation time: 10 minutes

Cooking time: 14 minutes

Servings: 2

Ingredients:

- 2 eggplants
- 1 teaspoon of vinegar
- 1 tablespoon of olive oil
- 1 teaspoon of curry powder
- 1 garlic clove
- 3 tablespoons of chicken stock

Directions:

1. Peel the eggplants and cut them into the cubes.
2. Sprinkle the eggplants with the curry powder and chicken broth.
3. Put the vegetables in the air fryer and cook for 14 minutes at 390º F.
4. Stir the eggplants every 5 minutes.

5. When the eggplants are cooked, allow them to cool in room temperature.

6. Sprinkle the vegetables with the vegetable oil and vinegar. Stir and serve!

Nutrition:

- Calories: 204
- Fat: 8.2 g
- Fiber: 19.7 g
- Carbs: 33.4 g
- Protein: 5.7 g

Cajun Spiced Lemon-Shrimp Kebabs

Preparation time: 5 minutes

Cooking time: 10 minutes

Servings: 2

Ingredients:

- 1 tsp. of cayenne
- 1 tsp. of garlic powder
- 1 tsp. of kosher salt
- 1 tsp. of onion powder
- 1 tsp. of oregano
- 1 tsp. of paprika
- 12 pcs of XL shrimp
- 2 lemons; sliced thinly crosswise
- 2 tbsp. of olive oil

Directions:

1. In a bowl, mix all ingredients except for sliced lemons. Marinate for 10 minutes.

2. Thread 3 shrimps per steel skewer.

3. Place in skewer rack.

4. Cook for 5 minutes at 390° F.

5. Serve and enjoy with freshly squeezed lemon.

Nutrition:

- Calories: 232
- Carbs: 7.9 g
- Protein: 15.9 g
- Fat: 15.1 g

Delicious Crab Cakes

Cooking time: 10 minutes

Servings: 4

Ingredients:

- 8 oz. of crab meat
- 2 tbsp. of butter; melted
- 2 tsp. of Dijon mustard
- 2 tbsp. mayonnaise
- 1 egg; lightly beaten
- 1/2 tsp. of old bay seasoning
- 1 green onion; sliced
- 2 tbsp. of parsley; chopped
- 1/4 cup of almond flour
- 1/4 tsp. of pepper
- 1/2 tsp. of salt

Directions:

1. Add all ingredients except butter in a bowl and blend until well mixed.
2. Make 4 equal shapes of patties from mixture and place on parchment lined plate.
3. Place plate in the fridge for 30 minutes.
4. Spray air fryer basket with cooking spray.
5. Brush melted butter on each side of crab patties.
6. Place crab patties in air fryer basket and cook for 10 minutes at 350° F.
7. Turn patties halfway through.
8. Serve and enjoy.

Nutrition:

- Calories: 136
- Fat: 12.6 g
- Carbohydrates: 4.1 g
- Sugar: 0.5 g
- Protein: 10.3 g
- Cholesterol: 88 mg

Crispy Fish Sticks

Cooking time: 10 minutes

Servings: 4

Ingredients:

- 1 lb. of white fish; cut into pieces
- 3/4 tsp. of Cajun seasoning
- 1 1/2 cups of pork rind; crushed
- 2 tbsps. of water
- 2 tbsps. of Dijon mustard
- 1/4 cup of mayonnaise
- Pepper
- Salt

Directions:

1. Spray air fryer basket with cooking spray.
2. In a small bowl, whisk together mayonnaise, water, and mustard.
3. In a shallow bowl, mix together pork rind, pepper, Cajun seasoning, and salt.

4. Dip fish pieces in mayo mixture and coat with pork rind mixture and place in the air fryer basket.
5. Cook at 400° F for 5 minutes. Turn fish sticks to a different side and cook for 5 minutes more.
6. Serve and enjoy.

Nutrition:

- Calories: 397
- Fat: 36.4 g
- Carbohydrates: 4 g
- Sugar: 1 g
- Protein: 14.7 g
- Cholesterol: 4 mg

Flavorful Parmesan Shrimp

Preparation time: 10 minutes

Cooking time: 10 minutes

Servings: 6

Ingredients:

- 2 lbs. of cooked shrimp; peeled and deveined
- 2 tbsps. of olive oil
- 1/2 tsp. of onion powder
- 1 tsp. of basil
- 1/2 tsp. of oregano
- 2/3 cup of parmesan cheese; grated
- 3 garlic cloves; minced
- 1/4 tsp. of pepper

Directions:

1. In a large bowl, combine together garlic, oil, onion powder, oregano, pepper, and cheese.
2. Add shrimp in a bowl and toss until well coated.
3. Spray air fryer basket with cooking spray.

19

4. Add shrimp into the air fryer basket and cook at 350° F for 8-10 minutes.
5. Serve and enjoy.

Nutrition:

- Calories: 233
- Fat: 7.9 g
- Carbohydrates: 3.2 g
- Sugar: 0.1 g
- Protein: 35.6 g
- Cholesterol: 32 mg

Shrimp with Veggie

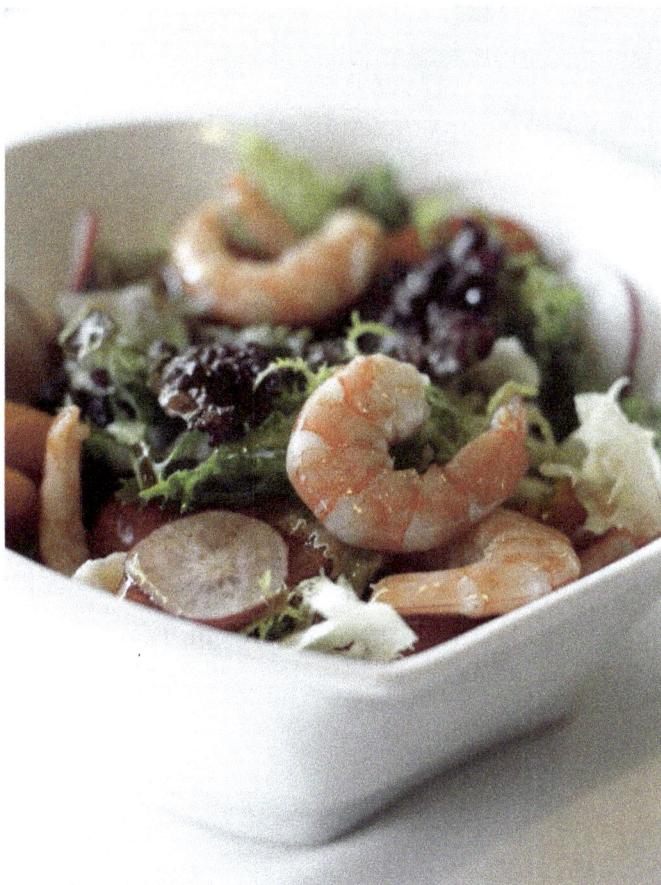

Preparation time: 10 minutes

Cooking time: 20 minutes

Servings: 4

Ingredients:

- 50 small shrimp
- 1 tbsp. of Cajun seasoning
- 1 bag of frozen mix vegetables
- 1 tbsp. of olive oil

Directions:

- Line air fryer basket with aluminum foil.
- Add all ingredients into the massive bowl and toss well.
- Transfer shrimp and vegetable mixture into the air fryer basket and cook at 350° F for 10 minutes.
- Toss well and cook for 10 minutes more.
- Serve and enjoy.

Nutrition:

- Calories: 101
- Fat: 4 g
- Carbohydrates: 14 g
- Sugar: 1 g
- Protein: 2 g
- Cholesterol: 3 mg

Simple Air Fryer Salmon

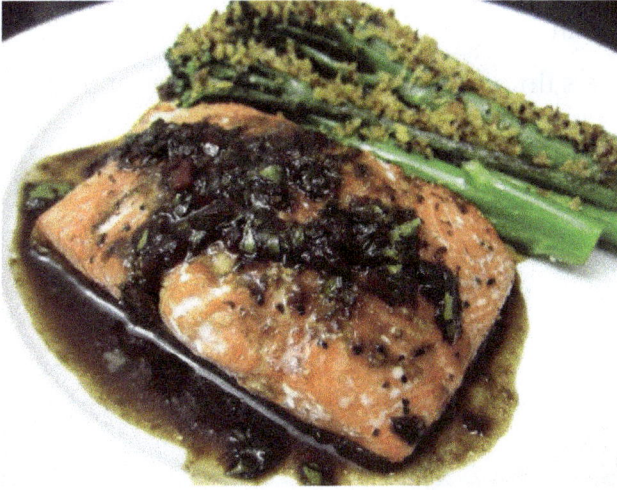

Preparation time: 5 minutes

Cooking time: 10 minutes

Servings: 2

Ingredients:

- 2 salmon fillets; skinless and boneless

- 1 tsp. of olive oil

- Pepper

- Salt

Directions:

1. Coat salmon fillets with olive oil and season with pepper and salt.
2. Place salmon fillets in air fryer basket and cook at 360° F for 8-10 minutes.
3. Serve and enjoy.

Nutrition:

- Calories: 256
- Fat: 13.3 g
- Carbohydrates: 0 g
- Sugar: 0 g
- Protein: 34.5 g
- Cholesterol: 78 mg

Cajun Spiced Veggie-Shrimp Bake

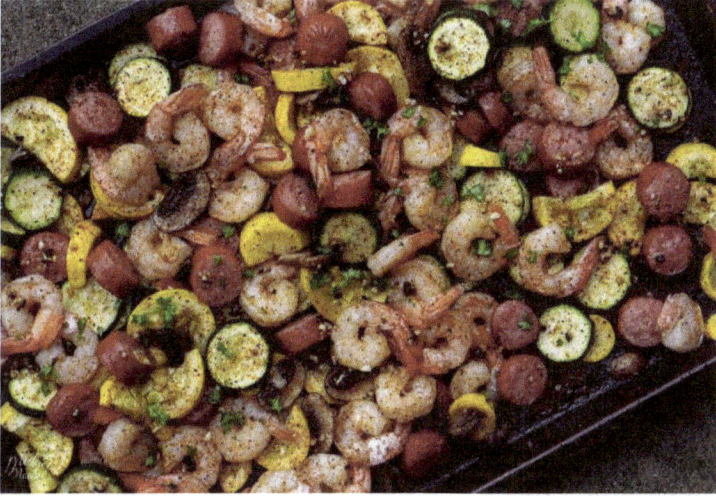

Preparation time: 5 minutes

Cooking time: 20 minutes

Servings: 4

Ingredients:

- 1 Bag of Frozen Mixed Vegetables

- 1 tbsp. of Gluten Free Cajun Seasoning

- Olive Oil Spray

- Season with salt and pepper

- Small Shrimp; Peeled & Deveined (Regular Size Bag about 50-80 Small Shrimp)

Directions:

1. Lightly grease the air fryer baking pan with cooking spray. Add all ingredients and toss well to coat. Season with pepper and salt, generously.
2. Cook on 330° F for 10 minutes. Halfway through cooking time, stir.
3. Cook for 10 minutes at 330° F.
4. Serve and enjoy.

Nutrition:

- Calories: 78
- Carbs: 13.2 g
- Protein: 2.8 g
- Fat: 1.5 g

Delicious White Fish

Cooking time: 10 minutes

Servings: 2

Ingredients:

- 12 oz. of white fish fillets
- 1/2 tsp. of onion powder
- 1/2 tsp. of lemon pepper seasoning
- 1/2 tsp. of garlic powder
- 1 tbsp. of olive oil
- Pepper
- Salt

Directions:

1. Spray air fryer basket with cooking spray.
2. Preheat the air fryer to 360° F.
3. Coat fish fillets with olive oil and season with onion powder, lemon pepper seasoning, garlic powder, pepper, and salt.

4. Place fish fillets in air fryer basket and cook for 10-12 minutes.

5. Serve and enjoy.

Nutrition:

- Calories: 358
- Fat: 19.8 g
- Carbohydrates: 1.3 g
- Sugar: 0.4 g
- Protein: 41.9 g
- Cholesterol: 131 mg

Tuna Patties

Cooking time: 10 minutes

Servings: 2

Ingredients:

- 2 cans of tuna
- 1/2 lemon juice
- 1/2 tsp. of onion powder
- 1 tsp. of garlic powder
- 1/2 tsp. of dried dill
- 1 1/2 tbsp. of mayonnaise
- 1 1/2 tbsp. of almond flour
- 1/4 tsp. of pepper
- 1/4 tsp. of salt

Directions:

- Preheat the air fryer to 400° F.
- Add all ingredients in a bowl and blend until well mixed.
- Spray air fryer basket with cooking spray.

- Make 4 patties from mixture and place in the air fryer basket.
- Cook patties for 10 minutes at 400° F. If you would like crispier patties then cook for 3 more minutes.
- Serve and enjoy.

Nutrition:

- Calories: 414
- Fat: 20.6 g
- Carbohydrates: 5.6 g
- Sugar: 1.3 g
- Protein: 48.8 g
- Cholesterol: 58 mg

Baked Cod Fillet Recipe from Thailand

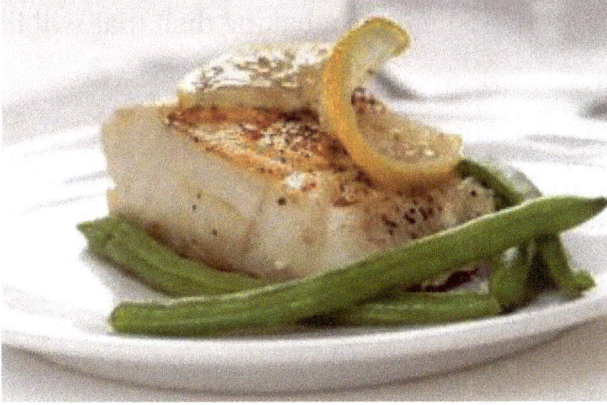

Preparation time: 5 minutes

Cooking time: 20 minutes

Servings: 4

Ingredients:

- ¼ cup of coconut milk; freshly squeezed

- 1 tablespoon of lime juice; freshly squeezed

- 1-pound of cod fillet; cut into bite-sized pieccs

- Salt and pepper to taste

Directions:

1. Preheat the air fryer for 5 minutes.
2. Place all ingredients in a baking dish that will fit in the air fryer.
3. Place in the air fryer.
4. Cook for 20 minutes at 325° F.

Nutrition:

- Calories: 844
- Carbohydrates: 2.3 g
- Protein: 21.6 g
- Fat: 83.1 g

Salmon Patties

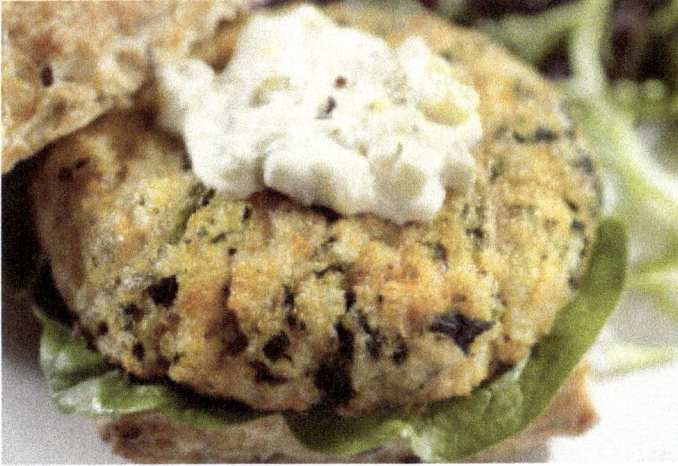

Cooking time: 7 minutes

Servings: 2

Ingredients:

- 8 oz. of salmon fillet; minced

- 1 lemon; sliced

- 1/2 tsp. of garlic powder

- 1 egg; lightly beaten

- 1/8 tsp. of salt

Directions:

1. Add all ingredients except lemon slices into the bowl and blend until well mixed.
2. Spray air fryer basket with cooking spray.
3. Place lemon slice through the air fryer basket.
4. Make 3 equal shape of patties from salmon mixture and place on top of lemon slices in the air fryer basket.
5. Cook at 390° F for 7 minutes.
6. Serve and enjoy.

Nutrition:

- Calories: 184
- Fat: 9.2 g
- Carbohydrates: 1 g
- Sugar: 0.4 g
- Protein: 24.9 g
- Cholesterol: 132 mg

Crispy Calamari

Preparation time: 5 minutes

Cooking time: 15 minutes

Servings: 4

Ingredients:

- 1 lb. of fresh squid
- Salt and pepper
- 2 cups of flour
- 1 cup of water
- 2 cloves of garlic; minced
- ½ cup of mayonnaise

Directions:

1. Remove the skin of the squid and remove any ink. Slice the squid into rings and season with some salt and pepper.
2. Put the flour and water in separate bowls. Dip the squid firstly in the flour, then into the water, then into the flour again, ensuring that it is entirely covered with flour.
3. Pre-heat the fryer at 400°F. Put the squid inside and cook for 6 minutes.

4. In the meantime, prepare the aioli by mixing the garlic with the mayonnaise in a bowl.
5. Once the squid is prepared, plate up and serve with the aioli.

Nutrition:

- Calories: 247
- Fat: 3 g
- Protein: 18 g
- Sugar: 3 g

Buttered Baked Cod with Wine

Preparation time: 5 minutes

Cooking time: 12 minutes

Servings: 2

Ingredients:

- 1 tablespoon of butter

- 2 tablespoons of dry white wine

- 1/2 pound of thick-cut cod loin

- 1-1/2 teaspoons of chopped fresh parsley

- 1-1/2 teaspoons of chopped green onion

- 1/2 lemon; cut into wedges

- 1/4 sleeve buttery round crackers (such as Ritz®); crushed

- 1/4 lemon; juiced

Directions:

1. In a small bowl, melt butter in microwave. Whisk in crackers.

2. Lightly grease baking pan of air fryer with the remaining butter. Melt for 2 minutes at 390 º F.

3. In a small bowl whisk well the lemon juice, wine, parsley, and scallion.
4. Coat cod fillets in melted butter. Pour dressing. Top with butter-cracker mixture.
5. Cook for 10 minutes at 390° F.
6. Serve and enjoy with a slice of lemon.

Nutrition:

- Calories 266
- Carbs: 9.3 g
- Protein: 20.9 g
- Fat: 16.1 g

Perfect Salmon Fillets

Preparation time: 10 minutes

Cooking time: 15 minutes

Servings: 2

Ingredients:

- 2 salmon fillets
- 1/2 tsp. of garlic powder
- 1/4 cup of plain yogurt
- 1 tsp. of fresh lemon juice
- 1 tbsp. of fresh dill; chopped
- 1 lemon; sliced
- Pepper
- Salt

Directions:

1. Place lemon slices in the air fryer basket.
2. Season salmon with pepper and salt and place on top of the lemon slices in the air fryer basket.
3. Cook salmon at 330° F for 15 minutes.

4. Meanwhile, in a bowl, mix together yogurt, garlic powder, lemon juice, dill, pepper, and salt.
5. Place salmon on serving plate and top with yogurt mixture.
6. Serve and enjoy.

Nutrition:

- Calories: 195
- Fat: 7 g
- Carbohydrates: 6 g
- Sugar: 2 g
- Protein: 24 g
- Cholesterol: 65 mg

Buttered Garlic-Oregano on Clams

Preparation time: 5 minutes

Cooking time: 5 minutes

Servings: 4

Ingredients:

- ¼ cup of parmesan cheese; grated
- ¼ cup of parsley; chopped
- 1 cup of breadcrumbs
- 1 teaspoon of dried oregano
- 2 dozen clams; shucked
- 3 cloves of garlic; minced
- 4 tablespoons of butter; melted

Directions:

1. In a medium bowl, mix together the breadcrumbs, parmesan cheese, parsley, oregano, and garlic. Stir in the melted butter.
2. Preheat the air fryer to 390° F.

3. Place the baking dish accessory in the air fryer and place the clams inside.

4. Sprinkle the crumb mixture over the clams.

5. Cook for 5 minutes.

Nutrition:

- Calories: 160
- Carbs: 6.3 g
- Protein: 2.9 g
- Fat: 13.6 g

Nutritious Salmon

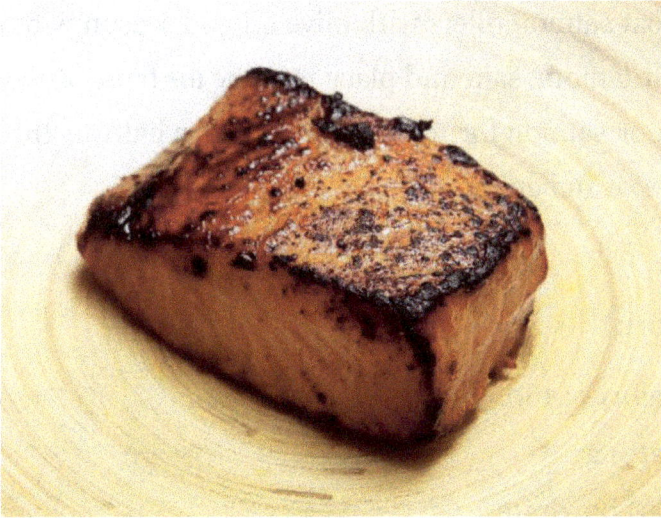

Cooking time: 10 minutes

Servings: 2

Ingredients:

- 2 salmon fillets
- 1 tbsp. of olive oil
- 1/4 tsp. of ground cardamom
- 1/2 tsp. of paprika
- Salt

Directions:

1. Preheat the air fryer to 350° F.
2. Coat salmon fillets with olive oil and season with paprika, cardamom, salt, and place into the air fryer basket.
3. Cook salmon for 10-12 minutes. Turn halfway through.
4. Serve and enjoy.

Nutrition:

- Calories: 160
- Fat: 1 g
- Carbohydrates: 1 g
- Sugar: 0.5 g
- Protein: 22 g
- Cholesterol: 60 mg

Almond Flour Coated Crispy Shrimps

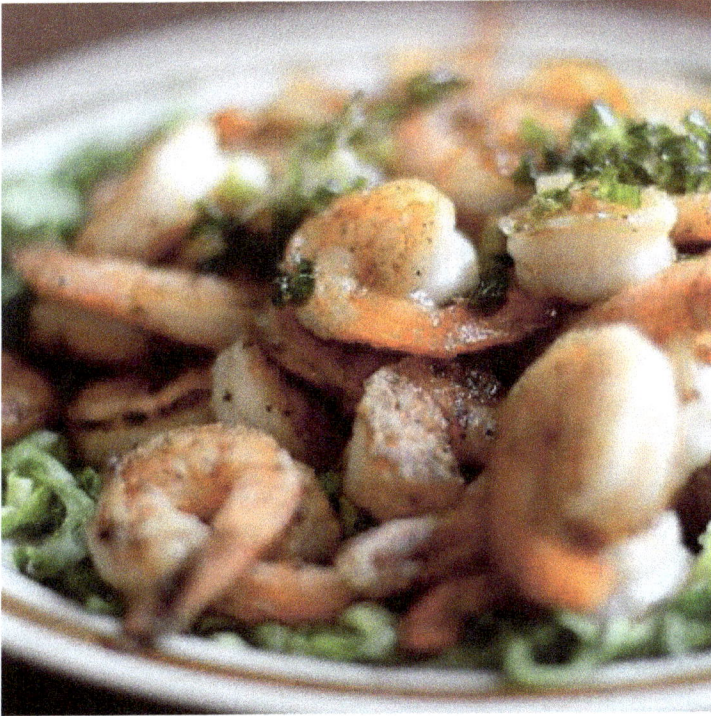

Preparation time: 5 minutes

Cooking time: 10 minutes

Servings: 4

Ingredients:

- ½ cup of almond flour

- 1 tablespoon of yellow mustard

- 1-pound of raw shrimps; peeled and deveined
- 3 tablespoons of olive oil
- Salt and pepper to taste

Directions:

1. Place all the ingredients in a Ziploc bag and give it a good shake.
2. Place in the air fryer and cook for 10 minutes at 400 º F.

Nutrition:

- Calories: 206
- Carbohydrates: 1.3g
- Protein: 23.5g
- Fat: 11.9g

Shrimp Scampi

Cooking time: 10 minutes

Servings: 4

Ingredients:

- 1 lb. of shrimp; peeled and deveined
- 10 garlic cloves; peeled
- 2 tbsps. of olive oil
- 1 fresh lemon; cut into wedges
- 1/4 cup of parmesan cheese; grated
- 2 tbsps. of butter; melted

Directions:

1. Preheat the air fryer to 370° F.
2. Mix together the shrimp, lemon wedges, olive oil, and garlic cloves in a bowl.
3. Pour shrimp mixture into the air fryer pan and place into the air fryer and cook for 10 minutes.
4. Drizzle with melted butter and sprinkle with parmesan cheese.

5. Serve and enjoy.

Nutrition:

- Calories: 295
- Fat: 17 g
- Carbohydrates: 4 g
- Sugar: 0.1 g
- Protein: 29 g
- Cholesterol: 260 mg

Lemon Chili Salmon

Cooking time: 17 minutes

Servings: 4

Ingredients:

- 2 lbs. of salmon fillet; skinless and boneless
- 2 lemon juice
- 1 orange juice
- 1 tbsp. of olive oil
- 1 bunch of fresh dill
- 1 chili; sliced
- Pepper
- Salt

Directions:

1. Preheat the air fryer to 325° F.
2. Place salmon fillets in air fryer baking pan and drizzle with olive oil, lime juice, and orange juice.
3. Sprinkle chili slices over salmon and season with pepper and salt.

49

4. Place pan in the air fryer and cook for 15-17 minutes.

5. Garnish with dill and serve.

Nutrition:

- Calories: 339
- Fat: 17.5 g
- Carbohydrates: 2 g
- Sugar: 2 g
- Protein: 44 g
- Cholesterol: 100 mg

Cajun Seasoned Salmon Filet

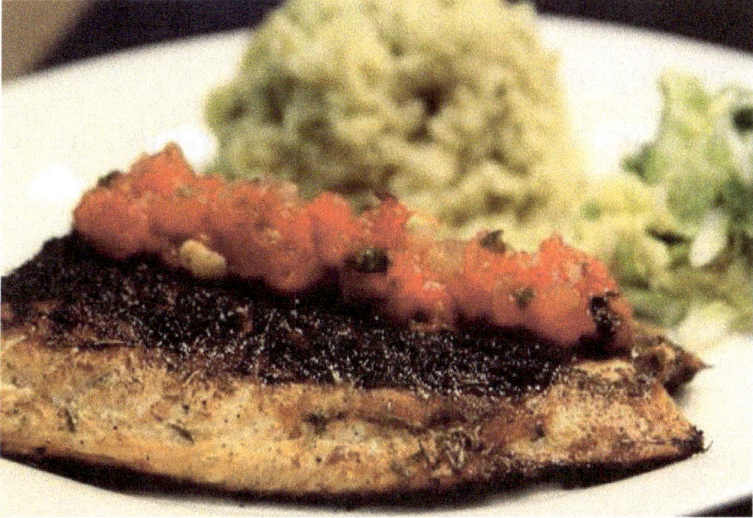

Preparation time: 5 minutes

Cooking time: 15 minutes

Servings: 1

Ingredients:

- 1 salmon fillet

- 1 teaspoon of juice from lemon; freshly squeezed

- 3 tablespoons of extra virgin olive oil

- A dash of Cajun seasoning mix

Directions:

1. Preheat the air fryer for 5 minutes.
2. Place all ingredients in a bowl and toss to coat.
3. Place the fillet in the air fryer basket.
4. Bake for 15 minutes at 325° F. Once cooked, drizzle with olive oil.

Nutrition:

- Calories: 523
- Carbohydrates: 4.6 g
- Protein: 47.9 g
- Fat: 34.8 g

Apple Slaw Topped Alaskan Cod Filet

Preparation time: 5 minutes

Cooking time: 15 minutes

Servings: 3

Ingredients:

- ¼ cup of mayonnaise
- ½ red onion; diced
- 1 ½ pounds of frozen Alaskan cod
- 1 box of whole wheat panko bread crumbs
- 1 granny smith apple; julienned
- 1 tablespoon of vegetable oil
- 1 teaspoon of paprika
- 2 cups of Napa cabbage; shredded
- Salt and pepper to taste

Directions:

1. Preheat the air fryer to 390° F.
2. Place the grill pan accessory in the air fryer.
3. Brush the fish with oil and dredge in the breadcrumbs.

4. Place the fish on the grill pan and cook for 15 minutes. Make sure to flip the fish halfway through the cooking time.
5. Meanwhile, prepare the slaw by mixing the remaining ingredients in a bowl.
6. Serve the fish with the slaw.

Nutrition:

- Calories: 316
- Carbs: 13.5g
- Protein: 37.8g
- Fat: 12.2g

Pesto Salmon

Cooking time: 16 minutes

Servings: 4

Ingredients:

- 25 oz. of salmon fillet
- 1 tbsp. of green pesto
- 1 cup of mayonnaise
- 1/2 oz. of olive oil
- 1 lb. of fresh spinach
- 2 oz. of parmesan cheese; grated
- Pepper
- Salt

Directions:

1. Preheat the air fryer to 370° F.
2. Spray air fryer basket with cooking spray.
3. Season salmon fillet with pepper and salt and place into the air fryer basket.

4. In a bowl, mix together the mayonnaise, parmesan cheese, pesto, and cover the salmon fillet.
5. Cook salmon for 14-16 minutes.
6. Meanwhile, in a pan sauté spinach with olive oil until spinach is wilted, or for about 2-3 minutes. Season with pepper and salt.
7. Transfer spinach to serving plate and top with cooked salmon.
8. Serve and enjoy.

Nutrition:

- Calories: 545
- Fat: 39.6 g
- Carbohydrates: 9.5 g
- Sugar: 3.1 g
- Protein: 43 g
- Cholesterol: 110 mg

Parmesan Walnut Salmon

Preparation time: 10 minutes

Cooking time: 12 minutes

Servings: 4

Ingredients:

- 4 salmon fillets
- 1/4 cup of parmesan cheese; grated
- 1/2 cup of walnuts
- 1 tsp. of olive oil
- 1 tbsp. of lemon rind

Directions:

1. Preheat the air fryer to 370° F.
2. Spray an air fryer baking dish with cooking spray.
3. Place salmon on a baking dish.
4. Add walnuts into the food processor and process until finely ground.
5. Mix ground walnuts with parmesan cheese, olive oil, and lemon peel. Stir well.
6. Spoon walnut mixture over the salmon and press gently.

7. Place in the air fryer and cook for 12 minutes.
8. Serve and enjoy.

Nutrition:

- Calories: 420
- Fat: 27.4 g
- Carbohydrates: 2 g
- Sugar: 0.3 g
- Protein: 46.3 g
- Cholesterol: 98 mg

Air Fried Cod with Basil Vinaigrette

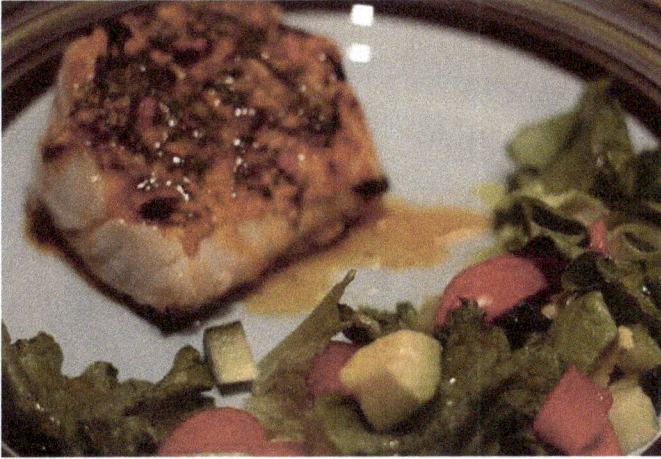

Preparation time: 5 minutes

Cooking time: 15 minutes

Servings: 4

Ingredients:

- ¼ cup o olive oil
- 4 cod fillets
- A bunch of basil; torn
- Juice from 1 lemon; freshly squeezed
- Salt and pepper to taste

Directions:

1. Preheat the air fryer for 5 minutes.
2. Season the cod fillets with salt and pepper to taste.
3. Place in the air fryer and cook for 15 minutes at 350 º F.
4. Meanwhile, put the rest of the ingredients in a bowl and toss to mix.
5. Serve the air fried cod with the basil vinaigrette.

Nutrition:

- Calories: 235
- Carbohydrates: 1.9 g
- Protein: 14.3 g
- Fat: 18.9 g

Lemon Shrimp

Preparation time: 10 minutes

Cooking time: 8 minutes

Servings: 2

Ingredients:

- 12 oz. of shrimp; peeled and deveined
- 1 lemon; sliced
- 1/4 tsp. of garlic powder
- 1/4 tsp. of paprika
- 1 tsp. of lemon pepper
- 1 lemon juice
- 1 tbsp. of olive oil

Directions:

1. In a bowl, mix together the oil, lemon juice, garlic powder, paprika, and lemon pepper.
2. Add shrimp to the bowl and toss well to coat.
3. Spray air fryer basket with cooking spray.

4. Transfer shrimp into the air fryer basket and cook at 400° F for 8 minutes.
5. Garnish with lemon slices and serve.

Nutrition:

- Calories: 381
- Fat: 17.1 g
- Carbohydrates: 4.1 g
- Sugar: 0.6 g
- Protein: 50.6 g
- Cholesterol: 358 mg

Filipino Bistek

Preparation time: 5 minutes

Cooking time: 10 minutes

Servings: 4

Ingredients:

- 2 milkfish bellies; deboned and sliced into 4 portions
- ¾ tsp. of salt
- ¼ tsp. of ground black pepper
- ¼ tsp. of cumin powder
- 2 tbsps. of calamansi juice
- 2 lemongrasses; trimmed and cut crosswise into small pieces
- ½ cup of tamari sauce
- 2 tbsps. of fish sauce
- 2 tbsps. of sugar
- 1 tsp. of garlic powder
- ½ cup of chicken broth
- 2 tbsps. of olive oil

Directions:

1. Dry the fish using some paper towels.
2. Put the fish in a large bowl and coat with the rest of the ingredients. Allow to chill for 3 hours in the refrigerator.
3. Cook the fish steaks on an Air Fryer grill basket at 340°F for 5 minutes.
4. Turn the steaks over and allow to grill for a further 4 minutes. Cook until light brown.
5. Serve with steamed polished rice.

Nutrition:

- Calories: 259
- Fat: 3 g
- Protein: 10 g
- Sugar: 2 g

Saltine Fish Fillets

Preparation time: 10 minutes

Cooking time: 15 minutes

Servings: 4

Ingredients:

- 1 cup of crushed saltines
- ¼ cup of extra-virgin olive oil
- 1 tsp. of garlic powder
- ½ tsp. of shallot powder
- 1 egg; well whisked
- 4 white fish fillets
- Salt and ground black pepper to taste
- Fresh Italian parsley to serve

Directions:

1. In a shallow bowl, mix the crushed saltines and olive oil.
2. In a separate bowl, mix together the garlic powder, shallot powder, and the beaten egg.

3. Sprinkle a good amount of salt and pepper over the fish, before dipping each fillet into the egg mixture.
4. Coat the fillets with the crumb mixture.
5. Air fry the fish at 370°F for 10-12 minutes.
6. Serve with fresh parsley.

Nutrition:

- Calories: 502
- Fat: 4 g
- Protein: 11 g
- Sugar: 9 g

Another Crispy Coconut Shrimp Recipe

Preparation time: 5 minutes

Cooking time: 20 minutes

Servings: 4

Ingredients:

- ½ cup of flour
- ½ stick of cold butter; cut into cubes
- ½ tablespoon of lemon juice
- 1 egg yolk; beaten
- 1 green onion; chopped
- 1-pound of salmon fillets; cut into small cubes
- 3 tablespoons of whipping cream
- 4 eggs; beaten
- Salt and pepper to taste

Directions:

1. Preheat the air fryer to 390° F.
2. Season salmon fillets with lemon juice, salt, and pepper.

3. In another bowl, mix the flour and butter. Add cold water gradually to make a dough. Knead the dough on a flat surface to make a sheet.

4. Place the dough on the baking dish and press firmly on the dish.

5. Beat the eggs and ingredients and season with salt and pepper to taste.

6. Place the salmon cubes on the pan lined with dough and pour the egg over.

7. Cook for 15 to 20 minutes.

8. Garnish with green onions once cooked.

Nutrition:

- Calories: 483
- Carbs: 5.2 g
- Protein: 45.2 g
- Fat: 31.2 g

Baked Scallops with Garlic Aioli

Preparation time: 5 minutes

Cooking time: 10 minutes

Servings: 4

Ingredients:

- 1 cup of bread crumbs
- 1/4 cup of chopped parsley
- 16 sea scallops; rinsed and drained
- 2 shallots; chopped
- 3 pinches of ground nutmeg
- 4 tablespoons of olive oil
- 5 cloves garlic; minced
- 5 tablespoons of butter; melted
- Salt and pepper to taste

Directions:

1. Lightly grease baking pan of air fryer with cooking spray.
2. Mix in shallots, garlic, melted butter, and scallops. Season with pepper, salt, and nutmeg.

3. In a small bowl, whisk well the olive oil and bread crumbs. Sprinkle over scallops.

4. Cook on 390° F for 10 minutes, or until tops are lightly brown.

5. Serve and enjoy with a sprinkle of parsley.

Nutrition:

- Calories 452
- Carbs: 29.8 g
- Protein: 15.2 g
- Fat: 30.2 g

Basil 'n Lime-Chili Clams

Preparation time: 5 minutes

Cooking time: 15 minutes

Servings: 3

Ingredients:

- ½ cup of basil leaves
- ½ cup of tomatoes; chopped
- 1 tablespoon of fresh lime juice
- 25 littleneck clams
- 4 cloves of garlic; minced
- 6 tablespoons of unsalted butter
- Salt and pepper to taste

Directions:

1. Preheat the air fryer to 390° F.
2. Place the grill pan accessory in the air fryer.
3. Place all ingredients on a large foil. Fold over the foil and close by crimping the edges.

4. Place on the grill pan and cook for 15 minutes.
5. Serve with bread.

Nutrition:

- Calories: 163
- Carbs: 4.1 g
- Protein: 1.7 g
- Fat: 15.5 g

Beer Battered Cod Filet

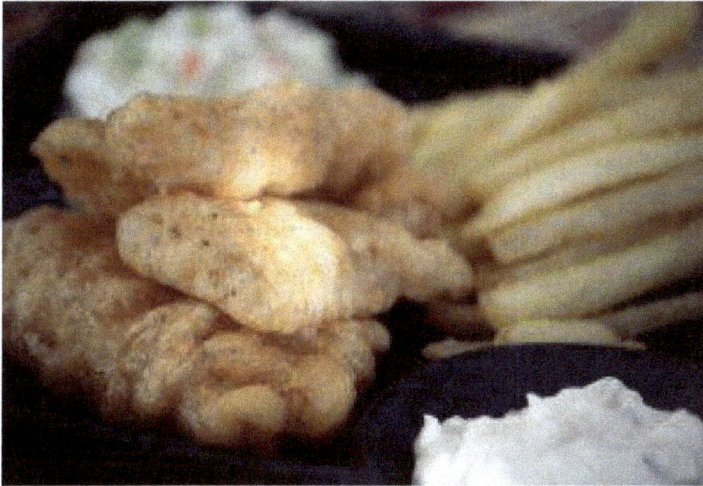

Preparation time: 5 minutes

Cooking time: 15 minutes

Servings: 2

Ingredients:

- ½ cup of all-purpose flour

- ¾ teaspoon of baking powder

- 1 ¼ cup of lager beer

- 2 cod fillets

- 2 eggs; beaten

- Salt and pepper to taste

Directions:

1. Preheat the air fryer to 390° F.
2. Pat the fish fillets dry then put aside.
3. In a bowl, mix the rest of the ingredients to make a batter.
4. Dip the fillets in the batter and place on the double layer rack.
5. Cook for 15 minutes.

Nutrition:

- Calories: 229
- Carbs: 33.2 g
- Protein: 31.1 g
- Fat: 10.2 g

Butterflied Prawns with Garlic-Sriracha

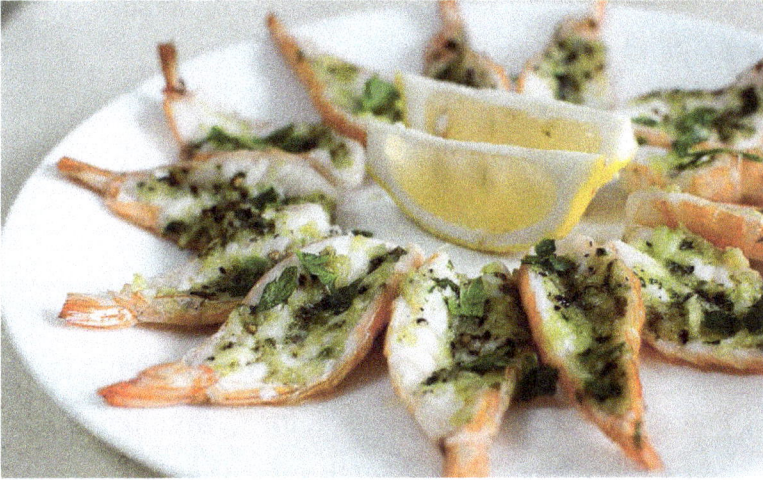

Preparation time: 5 minutes

Cooking time: 15 minutes

Servings: 2

Ingredients:

- 1 tablespoon of lime juice

- 1 tablespoon of sriracha

- 1-pound of large prawns; shells removed and cut lengthwise or butterflied

- 1teaspoon of fish sauce

- 2 tablespoons of melted butter
- 2 tablespoons of minced garlic
- Salt and pepper to taste

Directions:

1. Preheat the air fryer to 390° F.
2. Place the grill pan accessory in the air fryer.
3. Season the prawns with the rest of the ingredients.
4. Place on the grill pan and cook for 15 minutes. Make sure you flip the prawns halfway through the cooking time.

Nutrition:

- Calories: 443
- Carbs: 9.7 g
- Protein: 62.8 g
- Fat: 16.9 g

Bass Filet in Coconut Sauce

Preparation time: 5 minutes

Cooking time: 15 minutes

Servings: 4

Ingredients:

- ¼ cup of coconut milk
- ½ pound of bass fillet
- 1 tablespoon of olive oil
- 2 tablespoons of jalapeno; chopped
- 2 tablespoons of lime juice; freshly squeezed
- 3 tablespoons of parsley; chopped
- Salt and pepper to taste

Directions:

1. Preheat the air fryer for 5 minutes
2. Season the bass with salt and pepper to taste. Brush the surface with olive oil.
3. Place in the air fryer and cook for 15 minutes at 350° F.

4. Meanwhile, place in a saucepan the coconut milk, lime juice, jalapeno, and parsley.
5. Heat over medium flame.
6. Serve the fish with the coconut sauce.

Nutrition:

- Calories: 139
- Carbohydrates: 2.7 g
- Protein: 8.7 g
- Fat: 10.3 g

Arugula and Sweet Potato Salad

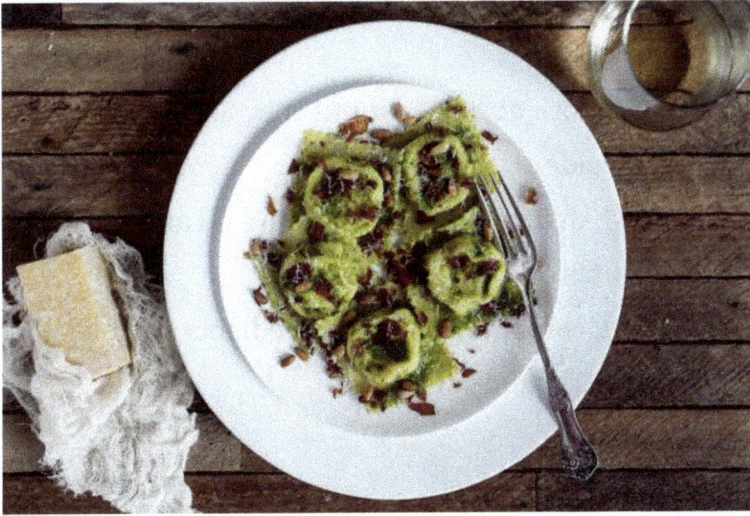

Preparation time: 10 minutes

Cooking time: 20 minutes

Servings: 4

Ingredients:

- 1 lb. of sweet potatoes

- 1 cup of walnuts

- 1 tablespoon of olive oil

- 1 cup of water

- 1 tablespoon of soy sauce

- 3 cups of arugula

Directions:

1. Bake potatoes at 400° F until they are soft, then remove and put aside.
2. In a bowl, drizzle walnuts with olive oil and microwave for 2-3 minutes or until toasted.
3. In a bowl, combine all salad ingredients and blend well.
4. Pour over soy and serve.

Nutrition:

- Calories: 189
- Total Carbohydrate: 2 g
- Cholesterol: 13 mg
- Total Fat: 7 g
- Fiber: 2 g
- Protein: 10 g
- Sodium: 301 mg

Nicoise Salad

Preparation time: 15 minutes

Cooking time: 10 minutes

Servings: 4

Ingredients:

- 1 oz. of red potatoes
- 1 package of green beans
- 2 eggs
- ½ cup of tomatoes
- 2 tablespoons of wine vinegar
- ¼ teaspoon of salt
- ½ teaspoon of pepper
- ½ teaspoon of thyme
- ¼ cup of olive oil
- 6 oz. of tuna
- ¼ cup of Kalamata olives

Directions:

1. In a bowl, mix all the ingredients together.
2. Add salad dressing and serve.

Nutrition:

- Calories: 189
- Total Carbohydrate: 2 g
- Cholesterol: 13 mg
- Total Fat: 7 g
- Fiber: 2 g
- Protein: 15 g
- Sodium: 321 mg

Scrambled Eggs with Goat Cheese and Roasted Peppers

Preparation time: 5 minutes

Cooking time: 10 minutes

Servings: 4

Ingredients:

- 1 1/2 teaspoons of extra-virgin olive oil
- 1 cup of chopped bell peppers; any color (about 1 medium pepper)
- 2 garlic cloves; minced (about 1 teaspoon)
- 6 large eggs
- 1/4 teaspoon of kosher or sea salt
- 2 tablespoons of water
- 1/2 cup of crumbled goat cheese (about 2 ounces)
- 2 tablespoons of loosely packed chopped fresh mint

Directions:

1. In a large skillet, heat the oil over medium-high heat. Add the peppers and cook for 5 minutes, stirring occasionally.

83

2. Add the garlic and cook for 1 minute.

3. While the peppers are cooking, whisk together the eggs, salt, and water in a medium bowl.

4. Turn the heat right down to medium-low.

5. Pour the egg mixture over the peppers.

6. Let the eggs cook undisturbed for 1 to 2 minutes, or until they start to set on the bottom.

7. Sprinkle with the chevre.

8. Cook the eggs for about 1 to 2 more minutes, stirring slowly, until the eggs are soft-set and custardy.

9. Top with the fresh mint and serve.

Nutrition:

- Calories: 201
- Fat: 15 g
- Cholesterol: 294 mg
- Sodium: 176 mg
- Carbohydrates: 5 g
- Fiber: 2 g
- Protein: 15 g

Marinara Eggs with Parsley

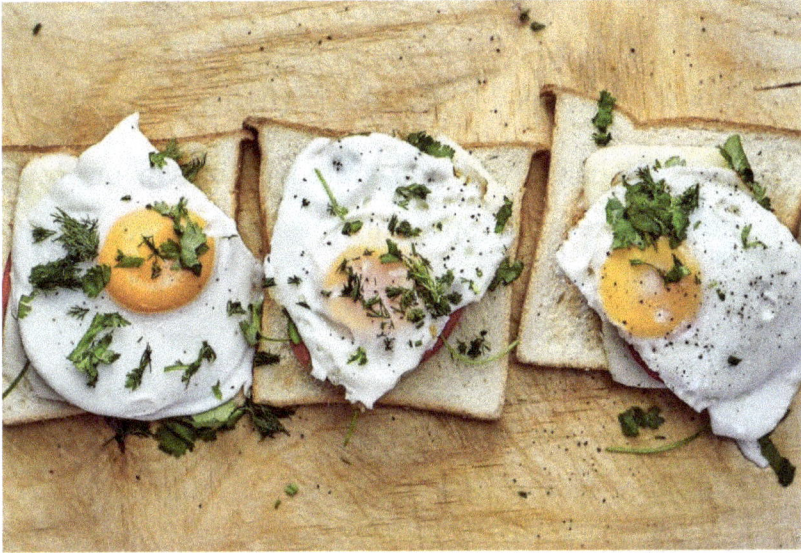

Preparation time: 5 minutes

Cooking time: 15 minutes

Servings: 6

Ingredients:

- 1 tablespoon of extra-virgin olive oil

- 1 cup of chopped onion (about 1/2 medium onion)

- 2 garlic cloves; minced (about 1 teaspoon)

- 2 (14.5-ounce) cans of Italian diced tomatoes; undrained, no salt added

- 6 large eggs

- 1/2 cup of chopped fresh flat-leaf (Italian) parsley

- Crusty Italian bread and grated Parmesan or Romano cheese, for serving (optional)

Directions:

1. In a large skillet, heat the oil over medium-high heat.
2. Add the onion and cook for 5 minutes, stirring occasionally.
3. Add the garlic and cook for 1 minute.
4. Pour the tomatoes with their juices over the onion mixture and cook until it is bubbling, or for 2 to 3 minutes.
5. While waiting for the tomato mixture to bubble, crack one egg into a little custard cup or mug.
6. When the tomato mixture bubbles, lower the heat to medium.
7. Then use a large spoon to form 6 indentations in the tomato mixture.
8. Gently pour the first cracked egg into one indentation and repeat, cracking the remaining eggs, one at a time, into the custard cup and pouring one into each indentation.

9. Cover the skillet and cook for 6 to 7 minutes, or until the eggs are done to your liking (about 6 minutes for soft cooked, 7 minutes for harder cooked).
10. Top with the parsley, and serve with the bread and cheese, if desired.

Nutrition:

- Calories: 122
- Fat: 7 g
- Cholesterol: 186 mg
- Sodium: 207 mg
- Carbohydrates: 7 g
- Fiber: 1 g
- Protein: 7 g

Buffalo Chicken Strips

Preparation time: 5 minutes

Cooking time: 25 minutes

Servings: 1

Ingredients:

- ¼ cup of hot sauce
- 1 lb. of boneless skinless chicken tenders
- 1 tsp. of garlic powder
- 1 ½ oz. of pork rinds; finely ground
- 1 tsp. of chili powder

Directions:

1. Toss the sauce and chicken tenders together in a bowl, ensuring the chicken is totally coated.
2. In another bowl, mix the garlic powder, ground pork rinds, and chili powder. Use this mixture to coat the tenders, covering them well. Place the chicken in your fryer, taking care not to layer pieces on top of one another.

3. Cook the chicken at 375°F for 20 minutes or until cooked all the way through and golden. Serve warm together with your favorite dips and sides.

Nutrition:

- Calories: 143
- Fat: 29 g
- Carbs: 15 g
- Protein: 30 g

Quinoa-Kale Egg Casserole

Preparation time: 20 minutes

Cooking time: 6 to 8 hours

Servings: 8

Ingredients:

- 11/2 cups of roasted vegetable broth
- 11 eggs
- 11/2 cups of quinoa; rinsed and drained
- 3 cups of chopped kale
- 1 leek; chopped
- 1 red bell pepper; stemmed, seeded, and chopped
- 3 garlic cloves; minced
- 1 1/2 cups of shredded Havarti cheese

Directions:

1. Grease a 6-quart slow cooker with oil and put aside.
2. In a large bowl, mix the milk, vegetable broth, eggs, and beat well with a wire whisk.

3. Stir in the quinoa, kale, leek, bell pepper, garlic, and cheese. Pour this mixture into the prepared slow cooker.
4. Cover and cook on low for 6 to 8 hours, or until a food thermometer registers 165°F and the mixture is settled.

Nutrition:

- Calories: 483 Cal
- Carbohydrates: 32 g
- Sugar: 8 g
- Fiber: 3 g
- Fat: 27 g
- Saturated Fat: 14 g
- Protein: 25 g
- Sodium: 462 mg

Chicken and Pasta Casserole

Preparation time: 15 minutes

Cooking time: 20 minutes

Servings: 6

Ingredients:

- 8 ounces of dry fusilli pasta

- 1 1/2 ounces of olive oil

- 6 chicken tenderloins, cut in bite-sized chunks

- 1 tablespoon of dried minced onion

- A pinch of salt and pepper

- A bit of garlic powder

- ½ ounce of basil; dried

- ½ ounce of parsley; dried

- 10 3/4 ounces of condensed cream of chicken soup

- 10 3/4 ounces of condensed cream of mushroom soup

- 16 ounces of frozen mixed vegetables

- 8 ounces of bread crumbs

- 1-ounce of Parmesan cheese; grated

- 1-ounce of melted butter

Directions:

1. Preheat oven to 400° F.
2. Lightly coat a baking dish with cooking spray.
3. Boil a large pot of salted water and cook fusilli noodles in it for 10 minutes or until tender but firm to the bite.
4. Drain water out of the pot.
5. Heat oil in a large frying pan on medium heat. Cook chicken in the oil with onion, salt, pepper, garlic powder, basil, and parsley for 20 minutes or until juices run clear.
6. Stir in pasta, soups, and vegetables. Pour the mixture into the baking dish.
7. Mix bread crumbs, parmesan and butter in a small bowl and cover the pasta.
8. Bake for 20 minutes or until browned and bubbly.

Nutrition:

- Calories: 416 Cal
- Carbohydrates: 33 g
- Sugar: 18 g
- Fiber: 15 g

Egg Mushroom Omelet

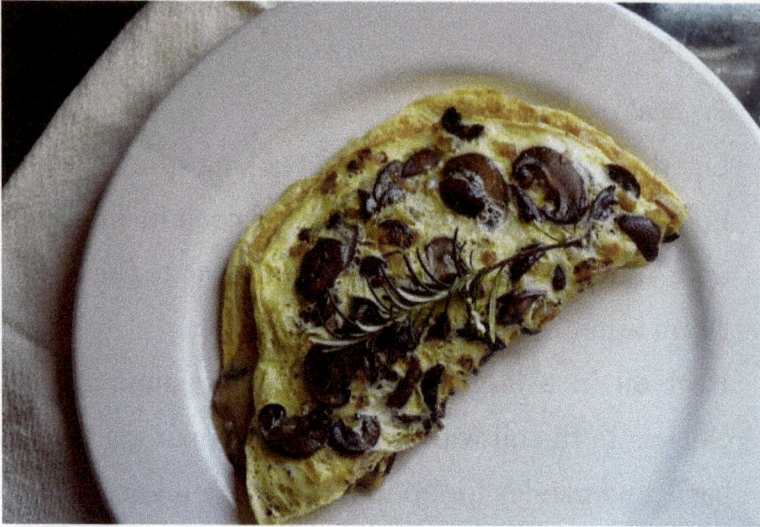

Preparation time: 5 minutes

Cooking time: 5 minutes

Servings: 2

Ingredients:

- 3 eggs

- 1 cup of button mushroom; chopped

- 1 baby shallot; chopped

- Sea salt to taste

- Cayenne pepper to taste
- 1 tbsp. of olive oil

Directions:

1. In a bowl, beat the eggs with sea salt and cayenne pepper.
2. Heat the oil in a skillet over medium heat.
3. Pour in the egg mixture.
4. Cook for 1 minute and add the mushroom and shallots.
5. Cover and cook for 2 minutes.
6. Allow to cool and serve.

Nutrition:

- Fat: 75 g
- Protein: 18 g
- Sodium: 195 mg

Egg Avocado Toast

Preparation time: 5 minutes

Cooking time: 5 minutes

Servings: 2

Ingredients:

- 2 almond bread slices

- 2 eggs

- 1 cup of avocado puree

- Sea salt to taste

- 1 tbsp. of almond butter

- Cayenne pepper to taste

- 1 tsp. of chives; chopped

1. **Directions:**
2. Toast the bread slices.
3. Spread the avocado puree onto the bread slices.
4. In a pan, add the almond butter and melt over medium heat.
5. Add the eggs and whisk for 1 minute.

6. Add the salt and cayenne pepper.

7. Scramble for 1 minute and add on top of the toast.

8. Add the chives, more salt, and pepper on top.

Nutrition:

- Fat: 18.2 g
- Carbohydrates: 19.3 g
- Fiber: 9.8 g
- Protein: 14.6 g
- Sugar: 2.9 g
- Sodium: 252 mg

Buffalo Chicken Tenders

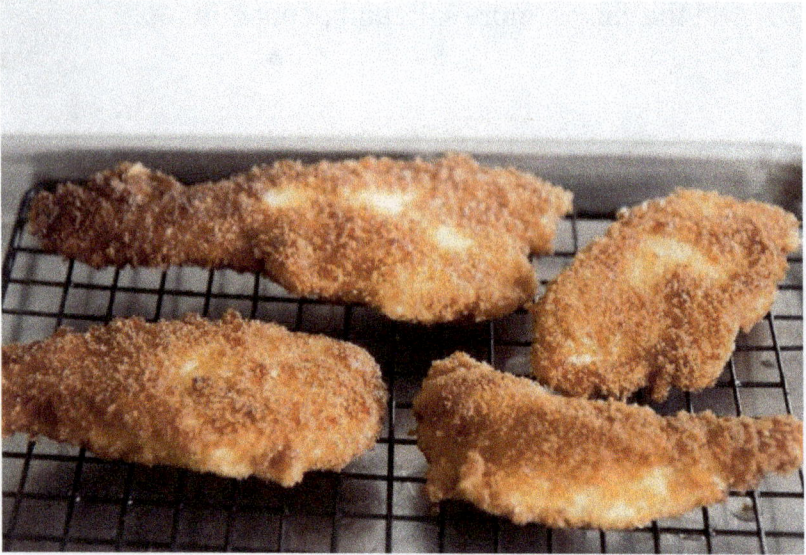

Preparation time: 12 minutes

Cooking time: 8 minutes

Servings: 4

Ingredients:

- 1 egg

- 1 cup of mozzarella cheese; shredded

- ¼ cup of buffalo sauce

- 1 cup of cooked chicken; shredded

- ¼ cup of feta cheese

Directions:

1. Mix all the ingredients (except for the feta). Line the basket of your fryer with a suitably sized piece of parchment paper. Lay the mixture into the fryer and press it into a circle about half inch thick. Crumble the feta cheese over it.
2. Cook for 8 minutes at 400°F. Turn the fryer off and allow the chicken to rest inside before removing with care.
3. Cut the mixture into slices and serve hot.

Nutrition:

- Calories: 240
- Fat: 10g
- Carbs: 20 g
- Protein: 20 g

Chicken Salad with Pineapple and Pecans

Preparation time: 10 minutes

Cooking time: 5 minutes

Servings: 4

Ingredients:

- (6-ounce) Boneless; skinless, cooked and cubed chicken breast
- Celery
- 1/4 cup of pineapple
- 1/4 cup of orange; peeled segments
- Tablespoon of pecans
- 1/4 cup of seedless grapes
- Salt and black chili pepper; to taste
- Cups cut from roman lettuce

Directions:

1. Put chicken, celery, pineapple, grapes, pecans, and raisins in a medium dish.

2. Kindly blend with a spoon until mixed, then season with salt and pepper.
3. Create a bed of lettuce on a plate.
4. Cover with mixture of chicken and serve.

Nutrition:

- Calories: 386
- Carbohydrates: 20 g
- Fat: 19 g
- Protein: 25 g

Crusted Chicken

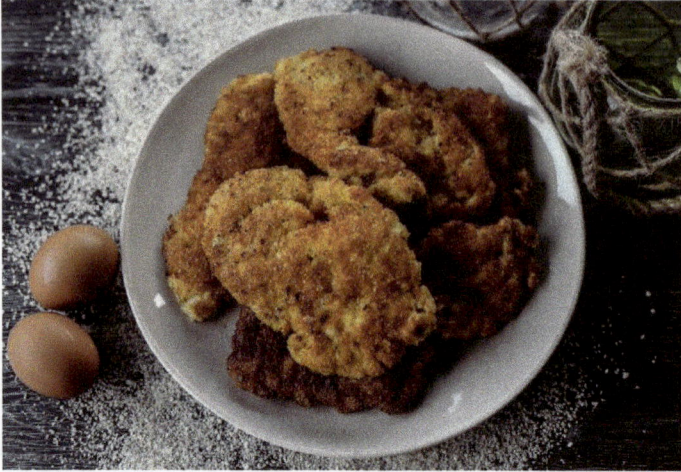

Preparation time: 5 minutes

Cooking time: 25 minutes

Servings: 2

Ingredients:

- ¼ cup of slivered almonds

- 2x 6-oz. of boneless skinless chicken breasts

- 2 tbsps. of full-fat mayonnaise

- 1 tbsp. of Dijon mustard

Directions:

1. Pulse the Slivered Almonds in a food processor until they are finely grounded. Spread the almonds on a plate and put aside.

2. Cut each chicken breast in half lengthwise.

3. Mix the mayonnaise and mustard together then spread evenly on top of the chicken slices. Place the chicken into the plate of chopped almonds to coat completely, laying each coated slice in the basket of your fryer.

4. Cook for 25 minutes at 350°F or until golden. Test the temperature, ensuring the chicken has reached 165°F. Serve hot.

Nutrition:

- Calories: 204
- Fat: 30 g
- Carbs: 14 g
- Protein: 23 g

Egg and Potato Strata

Preparation time: 20 minutes

Cooking time: 6 to 8 hours

Servings: 8

Ingredients:

- 8 Yukon Gold potatoes; peeled and diced
- 1 onion, minced
- 2 red bell peppers; stemmed, seeded, and minced
- 3 Roma tomatoes; seeded and chopped
- 3 garlic cloves; minced
- 11/2 cups of shredded Swiss cheese
- 8 eggs
- 2 egg whites
- 1 teaspoon of dried marjoram leaves
- 1 cup of 2% milk

Directions:

1. In a 6-quart slow cooker, layer the diced potatoes, onion, bell peppers, tomatoes, garlic, and cheese.

2. In a medium bowl, mix the eggs, egg whites, marjoram, and milk well with a wire whisk. Pour this mixture into the slow cooker.

3. Cover and cook on low for 6 to 8 hours, roll in the hay until a food thermometer registers 165°F and the potatoes are soft.

4. Scoop out of the slow cooker to serve.

Nutrition:

- Calories: 305 Cal
- Carbohydrates: 33 g
- Sugar: 5 g
- Fiber: 3 g
- Fat: 12 g
- Saturated Fat: 6 g
- Protein: 17 g
- Sodium: 136 mg

Egg and Wild Rice Casserole

Preparation time: 20 minutes

Cooking time: 5 to 7 hours

Servings: 6

Ingredients:

- 3 cups of plain cooked wild rice or Herbed Wild Rice
- 2 cups of sliced mushrooms
- 1 red bell pepper; stemmed, seeded, and chopped
- 1 onion; minced
- 2 garlic cloves, minced
- 11 eggs
- 1 teaspoon of dried thyme leaves
- 1/4 teaspoon of salt
- 1 1/2 cups of shredded Swiss cheese

Directions:

1. In a 6-quart slow cooker, layer the wild rice, mushrooms, bell pepper, onion, and garlic.

2. In a large bowl, beat the eggs with the thyme and salt and pour into the slow cooker. Top with the cheese.

3. Cover and cook on low for 5 to 7 hours, or until a food thermometer registers 165°F and the casserole is settled.

Nutrition:

- Calories: 360
- Carbohydrates: 25 g
- Sugar: 3 g
- Fiber: 3 g
- Fat: 17 g
- Saturated Fat: 8 g
- Protein: 24 g
- Sodium: 490 mg

Turkey Spinach Egg Muffins

Preparation time: 10 minutes

Cooking time: 30 minutes

Servings: 3

Ingredients:

- 5 egg whites
- 2 eggs
- 1/4 cup of cheddar cheese; shredded
- 1/4 cup of spinach; chopped
- 1/4 cup of milk
- 3 lean of breakfast turkey sausage
- Pepper
- Salt

Directions:

1. Preheat the oven to 350° F.
2. Grease muffin tray cups and put aside.
3. In a pan, brown the turkey sausage links over medium-high heat until the sausage is brown from all the edges.

4. Cut sausage in 1/2-inch pieces and put aside.

5. In a large bowl, whisk together eggs, egg whites, milk, pepper, and salt.

6. Stir in the spinach.

7. Pour the egg mixture into the prepared muffin tray.

8. Divide the sausage and the cheese evenly between each muffin cup.

9. Bake in preheated oven for 20 minutes or until muffins are set.

10. Serve warm and enjoy.

Nutrition:

- Calories: 123
- Fat: 6.8 g
- Carbohydrates: 1.9 g
- Sugar: 1.6 g
- Protein: 13.3 g
- Cholesterol: 123 mg

www.ingramcontent.com/pod-product-compliance
Lightning Source LLC
Chambersburg PA
CBHW062118040426
42336CB00041B/1848